Insomnia

Managing The Stress of Sleep Deprivation

The Grieving Heart Series

Aryla Publishing © 2018

www.arylapublishing.com
Visit the site for more information on books by Fiona Welsh
*and to be informed of **free promotions!***

Please see other books in my series

The Grieving Heart:-

How To Be Strong During A Break Up

How To Deal With Financial Stress

The Great Expectations Of Life

Rock That Body: How To Gain Total Body Confidence

Dealing with Death : Finding Your Way After a Loss

Depression: Dealing With Depression Mental Health Support

Anxiety: Dealing with Anxiety & Panic Attacks

Eating My Feelings: Control Stress Eating

It's Ok to Be Alone: Learning to Like and Love "Me" Time

Business & Home Series:-

How to Make Money Online

Keeping Your Children Safe

Table of Contents

Introduction

Certain medical words have been around for what seems like forever, but often get misused. For instance, the word 'stress'. How many times do you hear someone say 'oh I'm stressed', when in reality they're just a bit fed up or overwhelmed? Real stress isn't something to joke about, and real stress can be life-threatening.

The same thing can be said for the word 'insomnia'.

If you hear someone saying they are an insomniac, or they've got insomnia, the chances are that they just haven't slept well for one or two nights. Real insomnia? That's nothing to joke about at all.

In order to really highlight the importance of insomnia awareness, including its dangers and how it affects everyday life, we need to explore it in much more detail. This book is going to do just that.

If you have trouble sleeping on a regular basis, you spend your days yawning, feeling fatigued, never really having energy, and then dreading bed time coming around, because you know you're going to have to go through the whole restless rigmarole once more, you could very well be suffering with insomnia.

Insomnia isn't just one bad night's sleep, and it isn't just a little tiredness, it is a prolonged period of disrupted sleep, even no sleep, which causes all manner of upsetting physical and mental symptoms. Insomnia, real insomnia, is something to address and treat, to allow normal sleeping patterns to resume.

If you think you might be suffering from insomnia, this book is going to give you all the information you need to know about ways to treat it, where to get help, give you information about the condition overall, as well as help you understand the causes in much more detail. There is light at the end of the tunnel, but to get there, you first need to understand the condition you're suffering with.

So, let's address the actual definition of what insomnia is.

What is Insomnia?

The hard definition of insomnia is difficult to pin-point, but generally speaking, most experts agree that it is a difficulty in actually falling asleep on a regular basis, or a difficulty in staying asleep, even when there is no reason to wake up, e.g. no loud noise etc.

This lack of sleep quality can lead the person to wake up the next morning feeling literally like they have had no sleep, unable to concentrate, mood swings, feeling fatigued, and stressed because they know they're not going to be able to perform as well as they need to, e.g. at school or at work.

What sets insomnia apart from a simple phase of disrupted sleep and the actual condition is how long it actually lasts for. Acute insomnia is a phase which doesn't last for too long, but can be quite severe whilst its lasts. This is usually due to conditions in a person's life, e.g. stress or a negative event happening. In this case, once the issue resolves itself, the insomnia tends to resolve itself too.

On the other hand, chronic insomnia is a more ongoing problem. This is classified by sleep which is affected at least three out of the seven nights in a week, and lasts for more than three months in general.

You can understand how both situations can be upsetting and difficult to live with, but chronic insomnia is one which will cause the most negative effect in someone's life.

Insomnia tends to affect adults much more than children, and it is estimated that around 30% of the population is affected to some degree. That's a large chunk of people requiring help, so let's get onto the nitty gritty of the insomnia situation, and learn more about it, including where to get help if you need it.

Chapter 1: The Symptoms and Causes of Insomnia

Insomnia isn't simply not being able to sleep, it is about much more than that. Insomnia is a condition which can cause havoc in someone's life, and can actually cause illness in the worst case scenarios. Sleep deprivation overall is dangerous.

In this chapter we are going to talk about what insomnia feels like, the symptoms which lead to the diagnosis, and we're going to talk about the possible causes for insomnia too. The good news is that often by changing sleeping patterns and addressing the causes, insomnia often either goes away, or at least decreases in severity quite drastically. Having said that, we need to highlight the very real dangers of sleep deprivation too, to help give you that final push towards getting the help you need.

You don't need to simply live with insomnia, you don't need to put up with not getting enough sleep and feeling extremely rough for the following day. You can get your sleeping patterns back on track, you just need the right information to be able to do so.

What Does Insomnia Feel Like?

Most people with insomnia would agree that 'frustrating' is the best answer to that question. If you've ever suffered with one night of not being able to sleep, either not being able to get to sleep, walking up constantly, or waking up far too early, you'll know that it isn't a pleasant experience. Can you imagine that on a constant basis?

Many people who suffer from chronic insomnia are at a high risk of developing depression and anxiety too. This is because not being able to sleep plays havoc with your mood, and by not getting enough rest, your body is on the fast track towards all manner of different conditions. When your mood is low, you begin to worry. When you're not getting enough sleep, you don't feel like you can perform at work or at school, and yet again, you start to worry even more. This all adds up to a snowball effect, which can take you down some very dark roads indeed.

So, to answer how insomnia feels - exhausting, frustrating, stressful, upsetting, worrying. That list really sums it up. The thing is, everyone needs different amounts of sleep, and there isn't a 'one size fits all' answer to the question of how much sleep you really need. Just because you can get by quite easily with 7 hours per night, that doesn't make the person who needs up to 9 hours lazy. Our bodies are all hard-wired in a different way, and the amount of sleep we need varies.

On average however, the amount of sleep an average person needs can be classified as:

- 7 - 9 hours for an adult
- 9 - 13 hours for a child
- 12 - 17 hours for a toddler or baby

You can tell whether you are getting enough sleep or not, by how tired you feel during the day. If you're constantly tired, the chances are that you're simply not getting enough sleep.

Symptoms of Insomnia

If you've currently having problems sleeping, you might be wondering whether you have insomnia or not. Chronic insomnia is, as we mentioned, classified by at least three of your weeks' nights of sleep being disrupted. This is either by not being able to sleep at all, not being able to get to sleep, waking up several times, feeling like your sleep isn't that high in quality (e.g. very light sleeping), or waking up very early and not being able to get back to sleep, even though you have a good few hours left before your alarm goes off.

Acute insomnia is a response to a situation in your life, and this is much easier to identify and put right. Once the situation passes, you usually find that your sleep pattern also rectifies itself.

In order to be diagnosed with insomnia, apart from how long you've been suffering from the sleep disruption, you will have the following symptoms:

- You regularly find it difficult to get to sleep
- You regularly wake up several times
- You often lay awake at night, usually worrying about the fact you cannot sleep
- You wake up early, and you find it impossible to fall asleep again
- You feel very tired after you have woken up, and this continues throughout the morning - you basically never feel rested
- You can't take a nap during the day, even if you're very tired
- You are irritable and notice your mood swings quite easily
- You find it very hard to concentrate and focus on tasks
- You may find your appetite is affected, e.g. you don't want to eat, or you want to eat more, and probably the wrong kinds of foods - you are likely to crave high sugar or high fat foods

This is a very classic picture of someone with insomnia, usually the chronic type, and these symptoms can have lasted for weeks, or even months, before someone decides to seek out help.

What Causes Insomnia?

One person's cause can be totally different to the cause for another person. Insomnia is a very individual kind of deal, and as a result, it can be hard to pin-point an actual cause. What we can do however, is give you a general list of the most common causes of insomnia.

- **Stressful situations** - Stress doesn't always have to be a short-lived thing, it can often a chronic condition which builds up and lasts for a considerable length of time
- **Anxiety or depression** - Some people find it easy to sleep when they are in the midst of anxiety or depression, and actually sleep too much, but some find it very difficult to get to sleep, which worsens the entire situation ten-fold
- **Loud noises** - Not everyone can sleep easily, and noise from outside, even a small amount of noise, can be enough to put an already difficult sleeper into the midst of insomnia
- **Temperature** - Some people find it difficult to sleep is either too hot or too cold. This is a personal thing, as warm temperatures might be enough to make someone extra sleepy, but on the flip-side, they might have the opposite effect
- **Discomfort** - Changing beds, i.e. a new bed or staying somewhere different, as well as a new pillow, can bring on a bout of short-lived insomnia
- **Stimulants** - Anything which contains caffeine, e.g. coffee, cola, chocolate, anything containing alcohol, and nicotine are all known to boost insomnia and cause issues for problem sleepers. Recreational drugs are also known to bring on insomnia and make the situation a million times worse
- **Jet lag** - An upset body clock can send you out of whack for a considerable length of time, and this will need to be reset, in order for the situation to right itself. Long haul journeys are

well known for their after effects, and insomnia is one of them

- **Shift patterns** - Similar to jet lag in many ways, insomnia can be brought on by changes in shift patterns, i.e. working nights then days, and swapping back around. Those who work shifts often suffer with insomnia to some degree and this can be very difficult to work around
- **Certain mental health disorders** - Schizophrenia and bipolar are two conditions which are known to affect sleep patterns and cause insomnia. The medications which are taken for the disorders are also insomnia boosters, which creates a rather large and vicious circle. In addition, Alzheimer's and Parkinson's are also known to cause insomnia, as well as an overactive thyroid (hyperthyroidism), and restless legs syndrome

The good news is that insomnia isn't a particular condition which can't be solved, and it's really down to the eliminating the causes, changing your sleeping habits, and that should right the issue. If you are taking certain medications for a condition, such as Alzheimer's or Schizophrenia, and it is severely affecting your sleep and causing you to suffer from insomnia regularly, then you should talk to your doctor and look into alternatives, or perhaps additional medications, to help you right your sleep pattern and get the rest you need.

Chapter 2: The Effects of Insomnia

We've established that insomnia is more than just feeling tired and not being able to get a good night's sleep every single night, and we know that it can affect life to a high degree, but how exactly does it affect health in general, your mental health, and your relationships with your loved ones? Let's explore in a little more detail.

The Effects of Insomnia on General Health

The effects of insomnia are basically the same as the effects of sleep deprivation. Over time, the less sleep you get, the more serious the situation becomes. The more tired you feel, the more irritable you get, the more prone you are to having an accident, due to total over-tiredness.

These effects can be separated up into various sections, but when we mention general health, we are talking about the body.

Insomnia can:

- Affect your immune system
- Increase blood pressure - an issue if you already have high blood pressure anyway
- Increases your risk of developing diabetes
- Can cause weight gain, which has many associated risks, as well as the potential for obesity
- Puts you at a higher risk of having an accident, due to extreme tiredness, which could obviously cause serious injury, illness, or even death

The risks of insomnia are probably much more towards the mental health side of things, as we are going to explore shortly, but that doesn't mean that there aren't certain risks to the body too. The risk of an injury, because you're simply far too tired to concentrate on what you're doing, could result in death. There isn't anything more serious than that, let's face it.

The Effects of Insomnia on Your Mental Health

Mental health takes a serious hit when it comes to not getting enough sleep over a long period of time, and the longer it goes on for, the more concerning it will all become. You run the risk of anxiety and depression if you don't sleep over time, because your body will become so low on energy, and your happy hormones depleted, that you simply won't be able to recover before the next day starts. It's a slow decline which you probably won't even realise at first.

Aside from heightening your risk of anxiety and depression, what other effects does insomnia have on your mental health?

Insomnia can:

- Affect your long term and short term memory, increasing your risk of memory-related conditions in later life
- Affect your focus and concentration, making work very difficult indeed
- Cause mood swings, being over-emotional, and irritable - This can affect your relationships, and also put you on that route towards anxiety and depression, as we mentioned before
- Affect balance, which increases your risk of a fall
- Affect sex drive, which could damage your relationships over time

The effects of insomnia on your mental health are not particularly positive in any way, and will certainly worsen the longer it goes on for.

The Effects of Your Insomnia on Loved Ones

Of course, whenever a condition affects your life, it will have an impact on the lives of those close to you, because your mood will change, and the way you interact with them will also become different. For instance, we mentioned in our mental health section that insomnia can cause problems with sex drive. Whilst your partner might be very understanding, can you imagine a partner who isn't interested in intimacy for a long period of time? Of course, it is going to damage your closeness and your relationship, and in the worst cases, it could cause a split.

In addition, you're going to be grumpy and irritable the longer your insomnia goes on for. Being short-tempered not going to make you the most popular person around, and it could also cause issues for you at work. For instance, if you are constantly snapping at people, not being very helpful, purely because you're so tired, how can you expect to develop and maintain relationships? It's impossible.

Over time, it could very well be that those you love will become rather fed up with the treatment they are receiving. Of course, that doesn't mean that you mean to upset people and push them away, but you probably won't even realise you're doing it. Splits with those you love, difficulties at work, and your friends suddenly deciding to go AWOL on you, these are all very possible issues with an insomnia problem, when it simply becomes too much for those who have stuck with you over time.

This chapter is designed to show you the severity of insomnia. This isn't simply not being able to sleep for a while, or having a few 'tossing and turning' nights, it is a serious condition which can lead to much more severe conditions down the road.

Chapter 3: Diagnosis and Treatment of Insomnia

We've talked about what insomnia is and we've discussed why it is a troublesome condition, now it's time to get practical! By this point, we are assuming that you yourself are suffering from insomnia, or you think you might be. In that case, you need to do something about it before it becomes a real chronic problem.

So, what is your first step?

First things first, you need a firm diagnosis.

First Steps to Diagnosis

Go and see your doctor and explain your problem. He or she will take a detailed history and they will also ask you about any issues that you have currently going on in your life. This will help them identify whether your problem is an acute insomnia issue, or whether it is more chronic, i.e. it has been going on for a longer period of time, and isn't really associated with events.

You should certainly check in with your doctor in the following circumstances:

- If you have had sleeping issues for a while and you have tried to change your habits, e.g. change the temperature in the room, relax more, and it hasn't helped
- The length of time your sleeping issue has been going on, has been spanning over a few months
- Your lack of sleep is affecting your life negatively, and you're finding it difficult to cope

These are basically the red flags which should lead you to your doctor's office.

Your doctor will then try and find out what is causing your insomnia, because that is the route towards treatment. If your particular doctor feels that it is your habits and thoughts which are causing the issue, you may be referred for CBT, or Cognitive Behavioural Therapy. This is a form of counselling and therapy which can help you change your mind-set and thoughts, blocking out unhelpful thought patterns, and focusing instead on the ones which will lead you where you need to go, i.e. to sleep!

It's very unlikely that your doctor will prescribe sleeping pills for you, because of the common side effects which are associated with these tablets. Once upon a time, these used to be the go-to treatment option, but times have changed, and we are now much more rehearsed in how to effectively treat sleep disorders. Aside from anything, sleeping pills are also very addictive, and it isn't unheard of to become seriously hooked on them. The only circumstances in which sleeping pills are ever prescribed these days are if the insomnia is extremely severe, or if other options for treatment have all been tried and failed.

Another route which your doctor might like to consider is referring you to a sleep clinic for further tests. This will help him or her come to a solid reason for your insomnia, which can then give better guidance on how to treat it.

Insomnia Testing & Sleep Clinics

Your doctor may decide to refer you to a sleep clinic. This is a specialised clinic which deals with sleep disorders, such as insomnia and sleep apnoea. The reason for this is because these conditions are very difficult to assess whilst the patient is awake, and they need to be sleeping in order for the professional to be able to look at what is going on, and how severe it is.

These types of clinics are not really like regular hospitals, and they are designed to look more like hotels or bedrooms, to help the patient fall asleep much faster, and for the assessment to take place. Having said that, this is still a clinic underneath it all, and there is a lot of highly specialised laboratory equipment in there, to help assess what is going on.

You will be encouraged to make yourself comfortable, and obviously try to fall asleep. You will be in a comfortable bed, and it will almost be like being at home, but you will be attached to various monitors, which assess your brain activity, your body movements whilst sleeping, the rate of your eye movements, and your heart rate. In the case of snoring and sleep apnoea, this is also assessed for further information.

Sleep labs are really a very specialised diagnosis tool for doctors, but they are unfortunately not that common and in quite short supply. Your doctor may refer you to a specialised centre such as this, but do bear in mind that the waiting time to be seen could be long. You could therefore decide to go to a private sleep clinic, but you will need to pay for this, and sometimes the cost can be high.

It's likely that you will be asked to keep a diary of your sleep patterns for a couple of weeks or a month before your appointment at the sleep clinic. This means you need to write down the times you went to bed, the times you got up, the rough time it took you to fall asleep and the time you woke up. You should also try and document the number of times you woke up. This will all give the technicians at the sleep lab more information to work with, and this can be compared to the information your sleep studies give when you're actually there and being assessed.

Medical Treatment of Insomnia

Of course, like most things in the world these days, there are medical routes you can go down to help treat your insomnia, as well as herbal and self-help techniques. We are going to talk about self-help techniques and holistic types of treatment in a later chapter, but for now we need to focus on medical treatments.

You can go to one of two places to for medications for your insomnia - a pharmacy or your doctor. It is always best to go to your doctor first and foremost, because he or she knows your medical history, and they can look into the problem in a much deeper way, whilst also looking for any possible interactions with the medications you're already taking.

The types of medications which you can take for insomnia (by prescription) include Benzodiazepine Hypnotics, Non-Benzodiazepine Hypnotics, and another type of drug called a Melatonin Receptor Agonist. All of these medications include a certain amount of sedative, and for that reason, you should be very careful when operating heavy machinery or driving after you have taken one of these tablets. The likelihood is that you will take it an hour or so before bed, and you'll find that your body relaxes, your mind does the same, and sleep will come much more naturally. Yes, these are a version of a sleeping pill, so you should be extremely careful with dosage, and always take them as recommended by your doctor only.

If you can try and manage your insomnia without medications that is always going to be the best route to go down. Medications for sleep problems are often laden with side effects, as well as the very real possibility of becoming addicted. If you can manage it in a more holistic way, that is always going to be a better option for you. If you feel you need medication in the short term however, speak to your doctor about the best option for you.

Non-Medical Treatments For Insomnia

There are of course many other treatments you can opt for when it comes to insomnia, which don't involve taking a tablet. We're going to talk about self-help and herbal remedies shortly, but there are a few physiological and mind-set training options you can look into too. These have been shown to be highly effective, and are often one of the first routes your doctor will refer you for.

Cognitive Behavioural Therapy (CBT) and Relaxation
The mind-set behind CBT is changing the way you think, so if
you have a certain mind-set towards sleep, e.g. you become
worried about going to bed at night because you think you're
not going to sleep, that therefore sets off a vicious circle of
events. CBT can help you to change that thought into
something more positive, which will help you to nod off much
easier of an evening.

CBT is a long and sometimes drawn out process, and
something which requires dedication and belief by the person
who is trying it out. If you don't really believe it's going to work,
then it probably won't for you. It's worth a try however, and you
should put your entire being into it, if you want it to work. You
will work with a trained counsellor to rectify your thought
processes, and he or she will give you various exercises to try,
which are designed to challenge your thoughts and rectify
them into something more positive and useful.

Relaxation training is another type of CBT method, as well as
stimulus control. Many of us are far too mentally stimulated
before we sleep, e.g. we check our phones constantly, or we
watch high action films before bed. Learning to be relaxed
completely and in that state of mind that sleep will come more
easily, is key. Stimulus control is also about teaching your
mind to recognise when it is time to sleep, via your
environment and how you set up your routine. This can often
be enough to help relax the mind and body at the right time,
and rectify a problematic sleep issue.

The great thing about these CBT and behavioural therapies is
that you can self-teach yourself to a certain degree, so you
can do them at home. Of course, you will need to be shown
the basics by a professional first, to ensure you're doing them
correctly. Relaxation training can also include something
called progressive muscle relaxation, which teaches the
person to tense and relax isolated muscles, bringing about a
sense of calm and relaxation. Breathing exercises and
meditation can also be equally as useful, and these are

options which your doctor could help refer you for. Meditation is also something you can try yourself at home.

Many people struggle with meditation at first, because they don't actually believe it is going to work for them. It's about giving it a go, but in order to do that, you need to commit to it. A little like CBT in general, you have to believe it is going to work.

A very basic meditation exercise goes a little like this:

- Settle yourself somewhere quiet, where you're not going to be disturbed
- Pick just before bed, as this is when you want to be as relaxed as possible
- Turn off your phone and close the curtains, make sure the room is dark and cool/warm, just as you feel comfortable
- Make yourself comfortable in terms of where you are sitting or laying. Have plenty of pillows and blankets, and make sure you aren't going to be sat awkwardly
- Close your eyes and concentrate on your breathing. Allow your breath to flow inwards through your nose for a count of ten, and then hold for five seconds. Then, exhale slowly through your mouth for another count of ten
- Repeat this process until you notice that your thoughts are beginning to slow
- Any thoughts that flow into your mind, allow them to do so, by simply acknowledging their presence, and then letting them flow back out the other side - don't bear them much air time
- After a short while, you will notice that your mind has quietened down, and your body feels heavy - this is the phase you need to be in
- Now, turn your attention to your toes - tense up your feet and hold for five seconds, before releasing
- Repeat this process for every major muscle in your body, from the tips of your toes, right up to the top of your head - by the end of this process, you will be feeling totally relaxed

It might take some practice to get it right, and that's perfectly okay. You cannot be expected to master the art of meditation from the first go!

As you can see, there is a lot of help at hand for insomnia, and lots of treatment options to look into. It's really about finding the right type for you, but medical and non-medical options have certainly proven to be very effective for many insomnia sufferers in the past.

Chapter 4: Self-Help and Herbal Remedies to Help Insomnia

In our last chapter we talked about medical and non-medical ways to treat insomnia, and in this chapter we are going to focus more on the self-help and herbal methods which are highly effective in their own right.

Of course, we should exercise a word of caution here - never start taking a herbal remedy on your own steam. Always check with your doctor first, especially if you are taking any other medications already. These can sometimes interact and render your medications either totally null and void, or much less effective. It's always the best option to check things out before you begin. If you get the green light, which is probably likely in most cases, then you are more than welcome to try the many herbal remedies for insomnia.

Firstly however, let's talk about the more routine self-help methods you can look into. These range from meditation, a little like we talked about in our last chapter, to more general topics, such as relaxing before bed, having a warm bath etc. Some things might seem simple, but they are super, super effective!

Let's check a few out now.

Effective Self-Help Treatments of Insomnia

This really comes down to a range of dos and don'ts. You will find that changing your sleeping habits will probably bring about a big change in your insomnia severity. This is really best tried for chronic insomnia, and not insomnia which is acute, e.g. linked to a specific event, which is going to go away quite soon. Of course, that doesn't mean you can't give them a go! By relaxing your mind, you will be able to cast away many of your worries, and hopefully drift off much easier as a result.

Regulate Your Sleep Times

Try your very best to go to bed at the same time every day, and get up at the same time. It's best to go to bed when you feel tired, and not try and force yourself to sleep. By keeping a regular bed time pattern, you will find that you naturally begin to feel tired around the same time. This is ideal for getting your body clock back in sync, especially if you're working shift patterns, or if you have been on a long haul journey, which has landed you in jet lag territory.

Try Pre-Bedtime Relaxation
For the hour before you sleep, try and chill out as much as possible. Take a warm bath, read a book, and basically kick back and try and relax your mind as much as you can. By allowing yourself to relax, your body will release the relaxation hormone, called dopamine. This will help you fall to sleep naturally. Some people like to read a book, some like that warm bath, perhaps try some lavender in your bath, or try a warm glass of milk.

Avoid Stimulation Before Bed
Avoid anything which gets your senses on high alert. So, we're talking about social media, checking your emails, having any argumentative chats, reading books which grip you, or watching action films or scary movies, which have you gripped to your seat. You need to wind down, not get yourself more wound up!
Most of us are also guilty of keeping our phones beside our bed, just in case someone wants to call or a notification from Facebook or Twitter pings in. Don't do this! Turn your phone to silent. Don't worry, your alarm will still sound!

Create a Sleep-Worthy Environment
Make sure your bedroom is comfortable and set up for easy sleep. Make sure it is dark, very quiet, and properly ventilated. You don't want be too hot or too cold. Install thick curtains to keep the light out, especially security lights from outside which have a habit of creating a big chink of light right in the middle of your bedroom! You could also wear an eye mask or use ear plugs.

Get Plenty of Exercise

It stands to reason that if you get plenty of exercise, your body is going to be tired, hence bringing on a good night's sleep. Make sure you exercise during days times on a regular basis, but avoid evening exercise before bed, as that is just going to leave you with adrenaline still coursing through your body, and not creating the best atmosphere or conditions for sleep. The best rule of thumb is to avoid exercising for four hours before bed.

Think Comfort

If your bed comfortable? If not, change it! Your mattress needs to be comfortable, your pillows too, and make sure that your covers are just right - just enough, but not too much, and not too scratchy either. You also need to think about what you wear to bed - are you comfortable? Don't go for anything too restrictive, and avoid any materials which might irritate the skin. Think baggy and loose, comfortable, breathable, and don't always think about fashion!

Avoid Eating Before Bed

Try not to eat for at least six hours before you to go to bed. This will ensure that your body has digested its main meal and isn't going to leave you with bloating, indigestion, or heartburn. These are not going to help you sleep! In addition, avoid anything containing caffeine, as this is a stimulant, and will keep you awake, not help you nod off. Do not go for a coffee drink before bed, and if you really need something, go for warm milk.

Kick Your Pet Out of Bed!

If your pet sleeps in the same room as you, it might be a good idea to change that up and make them sleep in another room. If they are moving around, and you're sleeping lightly, you're probably going to wake up and then find it hard to get back to sleep. Obviously, if you have young babies who are sleeping in the same room as you, it's not possible to relocate them at this time, but for pets? Out they go!

Avoid Smoking

Smoking is bad for you on so many levels, but did you know that it can actually contribute towards insomnia too? The reason for this is because smoking, i.e. nicotine, is a stimulant, and the more you smoke throughout the day, the higher the levels you have in your body. It's a regular fact that smokers find it harder to fall asleep, they often wake up more often throughout the night, and their sleep pattern is disrupted as a result.

Write it All Down

One of the most annoying things about being on the cusp of sleep, only to wake right back up again, is due to thinking too much, or having too much on your mind. Stress is a big problem factor for disrupted sleep, and it's probably the case that you're lying there in bed, thinking about everything that has gone on throughout the day, and you remember things that you want to do the next day to put things right. You then start to panic that you're going to forget that one thing you've decided will rectify all your problems, and from there you don't sleep out of another worry. The answer? Keep a pen and paper at the side of your bed. When you remember something and you're sure you don't want to forget it, scribble it down and forget about it. Repeat this whenever something pops into your mind. Writing things down clears them from our minds, and allows us to switch off much more easily.

If you are someone who likes to plan, i.e. you like to have a plan of what you're going to do the next day, set aside some time earlier in the evening to note all these things down. That will be one less thing to think about.

Get up And Try Again

If you're finding it hard to sleep and you've been laying there for a while, with no sleep coming your way, don't labour over it. This will only make things worse. Instead, get up and do something which is going to relax you and make you tired without over-stimulating yourself. Read another chapter of your book, listen to some chill out music, or have a warm bath. Then, when you're feeling your eyes becoming heavier, try again.

Keep a Sleep Diary
A sleep diary isn't just to show a doctor when you want to show him or her just how difficult you're finding it to sleep, it is also a very useful tool in terms of identifying patterns. Write down what you did that day, what you ate, what you drank, the time you went to sleep, the time you woke up, and any thoughts or worries you had during the night. Let this diary run for a couple of weeks and then review it. Can you see any patterns? Is there anything in there which is recurring?

For instance, you might begin to notice that when you eat a certain food for dinner, even if you leave it six hours before sleeping, as recommended, you still find it difficult to get to sleep. This could be a food intolerance or sensitivity, which is affecting your sleep pattern. You might have a problem digesting that particular food ingredient, which keeps you awake with heartburn or bloating. You might not even notice this until you keep that diary and identify the patterns. Of course, if you go to see your doctor about your insomnia, that sleep diary will also prove to be very effective in terms of helping them see how severe your insomnia is, and for them to identify any patterns which are more difficult to spot to the untrained eye.

Recognise Your Stress Levels
We know that stress is bad, and we know that if you allow it to reach sever levels, you're going to run into serious health problems. The thing is, that could all affect your sleeping too. How stressed are you? Many people are very stressed without even realising it. When you function at a high level of stress for a long period of time, it becomes the norm to you, even though it's far from normal in reality!

Give yourself time to understand if you can truly, hand on heart, say that you are a stressed out individual. From there, try and understand how stressed you are. This will give you the tools to work towards reducing it all and hopefully that will also sort out you insomnia too.

Think about it this way - if your mind isn't relaxed enough to let go of everything that has happened that day, how are you supposed to sleep? It's borderline impossible. It's like going to sleep after an argument, or when you're very worried about something; you can't think of anything but that issue, and you're so emotional about it that your mind just won't wind down. When you're stressed, just as when you're upset, trying to focus on even the smallest of tasks can be a challenge.

Stress management will certainly help with your insomnia in this case. The basics of stress management include:

- Talk about the problem that is bothering you, no matter how insignificant you think it is
- If you need help, never feel like you're failing to ask - it's a strength to say you need help, because you can recognise the event, without trying to cover it up and probably dig yourself into a bigger hole
- Get plenty of exercise - this will boost your mood and help you keep things in perspective
- Eat healthily - eating too much of the wrong kind of thing isn't going to do much good for your digestive system, and it isn't going to create the most harmonious sleeping habits either. On top of that, you're not giving your body the fuel it needs to counteract stress, if you pack your diet with too much fat and sugar
- Try relaxation techniques - The same can be said for trying to fall asleep naturally, but if stress is your insomnia trigger, you'll find that relaxation works wonders

Most people who suffer from insomnia find that by changing their lifestyle and sleeping habits, the problem tends to right itself quite quickly. These self-help techniques aren't particularly difficult, but they do give you the tools to make effective changes to your routine. You will also see that most of these techniques are also healthy lifestyle techniques too, so not only will you be benefitting from better sleep, but you will notice you feel healthier overall.

Herbal Remedies to Try

Complimentary medicine, i.e. herbal supplements and remedies have long been an effective alternative route for many people suffering from various different conditions. Insomnia is certainly a condition which can be benefited from herbal remedies, however before you try any type of supplement or remedy like this, you should check it out with your doctor. We mentioned this warning in brief before, but it is so vital that we need to reinforce the matter. All it will take is a quick visit to see your doctor and explain your problem and what you're thinking of trying. From there, he or she will be able to give you a yes or no answer, as well as giving you advice on some of the best herbal remedies to try.

For completeness' sake, as we are discussing all different types of insomnia treatments, let's talk about some of the most popular, and most effective herbal remedies and supplements for insomnia.

Valerian Root
Many studies have been done into the effectiveness of valerian root in sleep issues, and they have all shown many positive results. Having said that, with any type of herbal remedy, it's difficult to say whether it going to work for every single person on the planet!

Valerian root can interfere with some other medications, so it is vital that you check with your doctor before taking this particular supplement or remedy. There are a few side effects to valerian root, but these should be minor, and should be weighed up in terms of pros and cons versus your insomnia.

Chamomile

We have all heard of the naturally sedative effects of chamomile, and it is regularly used for insomnia conditions. If you are allergic or sensitive to chrysanthemums or ragweed, you should steer clear, but other than that, chamomile is a useful herb. You can of course take it in a tea, or you can take a supplement. Many people use a spray mist on their pillow of either lavender or chamomile mixture, and this is breathed in, to give the same effects.

Lavender
Lavender is a very similar beast to chamomile, and has natural relaxation and possible sedative qualities. Lavender can be taken in a tea, a mist, or it can be used in massage using essential oils. This is a very effective and flexible herb to use, and isn't only great for insomnia issues, but also for anxiety and general relaxation too.

Miscellaneous Herbs to Try
There are various other herbs which have reputed sleep helping properties, including passionflower, hops, and even lemon balm. These aren't 100% proven just yet, but there is significant evidence to suggest that there may be a large amount of use in them. Whether you opt to try these or not is a personal choice, but do bear in mind that no herb is ever 100% proven to be effective for you as an individual. We are all different and we react to different remedies in different ways.

Melatonin
Strictly speaking, melatonin isn't a herb, but a hormone which is naturally produced within the human body, as well as in plants. Melatonin has a key part to play in sleep patterns and regulation, helping the body know when to wake up, in line with the regular body clock pattern. In addition, this particular hormone has been found to be useful in other conditions, such as potential heart problems, and helping with jet lag. The good news is that melatonin is therefore approved for the treatment of insomnia, and can be done via supplements.

Speak to your pharmacist about the best way to take Melatonin for you, but generally speaking, you need to ensure that you take the dose at the same time every day, in order for it to build up in your system and become effective. The actual dosage needs to be correct, because some supplements can actually raise the amount of Melatonin in your body a little too much! Speaking to your pharmacist will help you to find the right dosage for you, and also ensure that this type of supplement is suitable at the same time.

Acupuncture

Okay, so certainly not a herb or a supplement, but an alternative therapy method that has been found to be quite useful. There is no real place to put acupuncture on this list, so we'll place it here, to give you the right amount of information!

Acupuncture is a traditional form of Chinese medicine and is very useful in insomnia treatment. If you're not a fan of needles, perhaps this isn't the best route for you, but if you don't mind them and can tolerate them, then you may find good relieve from trying out this form of therapy.

Acupuncture involves small needles being inserted into particular pressure points of the body. Occasionally, certain forms of acupuncture will also include electrical stimulation at the same time. By stimulating these points, acupuncture is thought to allow the freer movement of energy, unblock any blockages, and allow sleep to occur in a much easier way.

All of these herbal remedies, and the occasional complimentary method, have been shown to have varying amounts of use when it comes to treating insomnia. You can certainly give these a try, provided you speak to your doctor first, and it may very well be that alongside certain sleep habit changes, you can solve your own insomnia problem quite easily indeed.

Chapter 5: You Are Not Alone

When you are in the midst a condition of any type, it can seem like you're the only person in the world who is suffering at that very moment. Of course, it's not the case with any type of condition, because there are probably millions of others worldwide who are in the same boat as you. Having said that, when you're tossing and turning at 3am in the morning, it can be a very lonely time indeed.

There are countless reasons for this, and we discussed many of them in our earlier chapters. The thing is, we can certainly put a lot of blame at the door of our busy lives when it comes to the reason why so many of us struggle to get a good night's sleep on a regular basis. We've talked at length about stress, but what about money worries? How many of us lay awake at night doing our sums, trying to make ends meet? Many people do! How many people lay there worrying about that 'what ifs' and 'maybes' in the world? Again, this is something we seem to be hard-wried to do these days.

Our busy lives affect the way we live, and they also affect the way we rest. It's not as easy as simply saying 'okay, slow down a little' because our jobs don't allow us to, and our endless to do list isn't going to get any shorter by simply chilling out and slowing our lives! It's a vicious circle in many ways, but in order to help you feel like you're certainly not the only one suffering from insomnia, these are issues which you can use to take to heart and reassure you in that regard. Of course, that doesn't help to solve it, but it might make you feel better in the here and now!

The Prevalence of Insomnia in Today's Society

Insomnia affects millions. To give you an idea, let's check out some statistics.

The University of Warwick discovered that 150 million adults worldwide report sleep issues on a regular basis. That's a huge amount of people tossing and turning every night, in fact it's around 30% of the world's population!

In addition, the following statistics might surprise you too:

- On average, we (the general population) sleep around 20% less than we did around a century ago
- One in every three people will develop insomnia of some description in their lives
- Stress and anxiety (either or both) is one of the main reasons for insomnia for Americans, with more than half of the population having trouble sleeping
- For reasons unknown, women are more likely to suffer from insomnia than men, with a twice as likely chance
- Although proven link, it is though that a predisposition to insomnia could be true, as around 35% of those suffering from insomnia have a history of the same within the family
- Those who suffer from depression are likely to suffer from insomnia at some stage too, with around 90% of depression sufferers reporting insomnia problems
- It is thought that an estimate 10 million US citizens use some kind of sleeping prescription drug
- There is a link between insomnia and weight gain and obesity, which also increases the risk of another sleep-related issue, called sleep apnoea
- A poll by the National Sleep Foundation showed that around 60% of people asked have reported driving and feeling tired, with around 37% of those having fallen asleep whilst driving at some point
- The number one reason for low sex drive is tiredness

Those facts and figures are really quite startling when you think about the huge problem that insomnia causes in today's society. The fact that many people admit to driving whilst feeling tired is worrying, and the number of those who admit to actually nodding off at the wheel is even more worrying still. The sheer number of people who need to use sleeping aid prescription drugs in the US highlights the issue to a huge degree, and the complications which insomnia causes, e.g.

potential depression and anxiety, weight gain, obesity, and possible sleep apnoea, are also something to bear in mind.

Now, by reading those figures, do you feel that you're still alone in your insomnia problem?

No!

Known Sufferers in The Limelight

Of course, the plight of celebrities is never far from our minds, but by knowing that some of our heroes and admired stars also suffer form the same conditions as us, can help us realise that they are just as human as we are, and that what we're suffering from isn't something we need to face alone. The following celebrities have admitted to insomnia in the past:

- George Clooney
- Michael Jackson
- Jessica Simpson
- Marilyn Monroe
- Madonna
- Miley Cyrus
- Heath Ledger

Of course, celebrities live lifestyles which are quite chaotic a lot of the time, with a large amount of travel, stress, and probably being away from family quite a large amount. These all tie in with the potential causes for insomnia overall, and highlight the regularities.

Whilst insomnia isn't something we generally talk about over dinner, you only have to do a straw poll of your colleagues at work, or perhaps those you meet up with for dinner on a regular basis, to find out who else in your social circle actually admits to having sleep problems too. It's likely that at least half of them will raise their hand on this, and perhaps that's a great way for you to find allies in your corner. Having an insomnia buddy can help you to talk about your problems, and can allow you to off-load any potential problems or worries which are causing your sleep issues. Whilst it might not help for everyone, it's certainly worth a try, right?

In our next, final chapter, we're going to pull everything together, but we're also going to give you some useful websites to check out on the subject. These sites can give you more self-help techniques, more background information, and can also put you in touch with professionals who can talk to you, if you feel you need extra help and support.

Conclusion

And there we have it, everything you need to know about insomnia. By this point, the hope is that you are feeling much more upbeat about things, and that you are reassured that you are far from alone.

Insomnia is no laughing matter, and whilst many people may lament the so-called fact they have insomnia, when they simply have had one night of broken sleep, it isn't a condition which should ever be allowed to sail under the radar. Sleep deprivation in any guise is upsetting and potentially very dangerous. Over time, that deprivation can turn into a serious matter, putting you at risk of accidents, stress problems, high blood pressure, and total lack of focus. A lack of sleep is also a fast track towards an increased risk of diabetes, and that isn't something that anyone needs to add into their lives unwittingly.

Whether you are suffering from acute or chronic insomnia, it's important that you reach out and get the help you need. The great news is that insomnia can be solved relatively easily, once you find a method which works for you. Don't be perturbed if you find that your first option doesn't work, and that you need to try something else - you will get there! Everyone is different, so just because hot milk and a bath before bed worked for your friend, it doesn't necessarily mean it's going to work for you. It's possible that you might need a little more help, perhaps even medically speaking, but if that's what your doctor recommends, then it will get you to the same stage in the end.

The By-Product of a Busy Life

The reason for your insomnia, i.e. the cause, could be something else entirely, but it can't be ignored that many people suffer from insomnia as a result of a fast paced life. When we're constantly stressed out due to work, money issues, relationship problems, and trying to juggle ten balls in the air at the same time, it's no wonder that sleep is one of the first things to give way. The problem is when that issue turns into something which is prolonged.

The pressure to do everything and succeed can be too much pressure for any single person, so if you find you are becoming negative affected by stress, stop if before it becomes a huge issue overall. Speak to someone, talk it out, solve any issues that are adding up to the problem, and put sleep at the front of your priority list.

We are often far too stimulated before we go to bed, and that doesn't help matters at all. Turn off your phone, or at least turn it onto silent. You're not going to miss anything on Facebook whilst you sleep! Avoid those over-stimulating films before bed, and make it your priority to relax with a capital R in the couple of hours before you sleep. Try your very best to maintain a regular sleep pattern, if nothing else. Going to bed at the same time every day, and waking up at the same time is vital for regulating your body clock and ensuring that you maintain the right kind of pattern. When your sleeping pattern is all over the place, your body simply doesn't have the first clue when it is supposed to close down for the night and when it needs to stay awake. Do your body a favour and maintain that rhythm, and you might just find that your insomnia problem disappears.

Of course, there are going to be times when you need to stay up late, perhaps for a particular function, or you're away on holiday, but the idea is that it isn't a regular occurrence, and that you have a general pattern which your mind and body are used to.

If you find your household is particularly chaotic, i.e. you have children, teenagers, and many people making a noise at various different times of the day, sit down and have a talk with everyone. The fact that you are missing out on sleep because of the acts of others isn't acceptable, and also, perhaps they're missing out on their sleep as a result too! A few rules about noise levels should be all it takes to right the problem. Also ensuring that your room is as comfortable as possible, the right temperature, and as dark as it can be, will help you in your sleep endeavours.

Helpful Websites & Organisations

The following websites and organisations are on hand to help you with any issues you might have pertaining to your insomnia. The UK helpline is also very useful for UK residents who are suffering with insomnia and simply don't know which way to turn. By allowing you to speak to a trained professional, you can obtain the help and support you need. Of course, a visit to your doctor is also vital, in order to identify the cause of your sleep problem, and help you put in place ways to solve it, either via medical means or by self-help routes.

Insomnia helpline (UK) - 020 8994 9874

https://sleepfoundation.org
https://www.sleepassociation.org
https://sleepcouncil.org.uk/where-to-get-help/
https://thesleepschool.org
https://www.sleepsociety.org.uk
https://www.mentalhealth.org.uk/publications/how-sleep-better?gclid=EAIaIQobChMIwbKkuIOa3AIVxkQYCh1CGA5JEAAYAiAAEgKIXPD_BwE
https://www.healthcentre.org.uk/sleep-disorders/find-associations-societies.html

All that is left is for us to bid you goodbye and wish you luck. Remember, there is a lot of help out there, if you only take the time and make the effort to reach out and grab it with both hands. Insomnia isn't something to be taken lightly, but it is something which is entirely beatable. Whether you choose the medical route, the self-help route, or you go for a mixture, it's entirely personal, but there will be a route there for you.

Happy sleeping!

Thank you for reading my book.
I would love it if you could leave me an honest review on what you thought of this book.

If you like to know more about my books and the opportunity to be notified of free promotions please visit Aryla Publishing website

Or follow Instagram, Facebook Twitter

Thank you

Please see other Titles from

ARYLA PUBLISHING

Childrens Books
The Body Goo Series
The Billy Series

Adult Books
Self Help Books
Diet and Wellbeing
Fiction
Comedy Books
Romance Books
YA Books

Other Publications

Eating My Feelings : Control Stress Eating
By Fiona Welsh (Self Help)

Eat. Cry. Laugh. Repeat.

If you catch yourself

- **Chomping down on a box of donuts to celebrate the latest pay check.**
  •
- **Draining a tub of ice cream after a fight with your significant other.**
  •
- **Staring into an open refrigerator whenever you're bored.**

then you just might be an **Emotional Eater.**

Most people who are overweight use food as a comfort and coping mechanism; and are often unaware of the contributions of emotional eating to their waistlines. When diet is regulated by moods, emotional eaters will often try to 'self-medicate', by eating to get rid of unpleasant emotions, rather than when they feel hungry. And so, it is often the case that when feelings and food become linked, a food junkie is created, and the world becomes a little bit heavier. If this resonates with you, then the information inside this book is perfect for you.

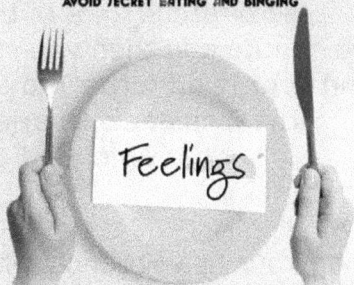

EATING MY FEELINGS

CONTROL STREET EATING WHEN HAPPY AND SAD, AVOID SECRET EATING AND BINGING

Feelings

Fiona Welsh

Anxiety: Dealing With Anxiety & Panic Attacks –
By Fiona Welsh (Self Help)

Do you regularly feel like you are always worrying about something? Do you often feel fearful? Do you wake up with a sense of dread a lot of the time? Do you feel fine one minute and then you start overthinking, and your mind turns into a hamster wheel of 'what if' situations and scenarios? Do you feel generally uneasy a lot of the time, and you can't really pinpoint a reason why?

If you are nodding your head to most of the above then it could very well be that you are suffering from an anxiety disorder.

Anxiety is more common than you might even think. It is thought that 1 in every 13 people will suffer from an anxiety disorder at some stage in their lives, and this equates to around 7.3% of the world's population. The statistics are startling, and that makes anxiety the most common mental disorder in the spectrum.

If you're feeling like you might have a problem with anxiety, these statistics should give you a little hope – you're not alone, you're not going crazy, the world isn't the dark place that you might be led to believe; there is help at hand.

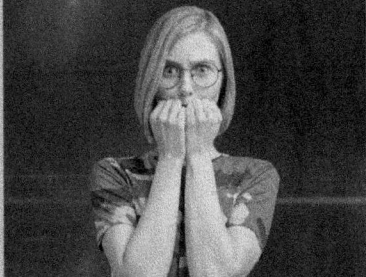

The Truth About Getting Old –
By Tyler Moses (Comedy)

Congratulations and welcome to the over 40s club!
You have worked hard to get to this pinnacle point in
life, so let's take a moment to celebrate being over 40
and everything that comes with it. Your body has been
through a lot in order to get you over the hill, and
your 40s is when some of your parts may start to,
well, retire. During your time in the old person club,
your body will experience new and not-so-exciting
changes around every corner (even though we take
corners slowly now as to avoid obstacles that may
knock us off balance). Grab your Biotene and a large
supply of antacids and sit back on your heating pad as
we journey into the life of being over 40.

THE TRUTH ABOUT
GETTING
OLD

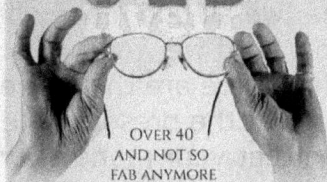

OVER 40
AND NOT SO
FAB ANYMORE

TYLER MSES

How to Make Money Online –
By Fiona Welsh (Self Help – Business)

Unfortunately, the pot of gold at the end of the rainbow is yet to be found, there doesn't seem to be a Leprechaun smiling at whoever manages to stumble upon this long-famed prize, and as for the money tree, well, it's still as elusive as ever.

From time to time, we all find money hard to come by, and no matter how hard we work, or how much we save, it's likely that there are things we want and need that we can't afford at the present time. Obviously, that doesn't mean that your money situation is going to be difficult all the time, because cash flow ebbs and flows (pardon the pun) as much as anything in life, but finding ways to help it along a little is always a good thing.

The internet has changed so much about our modern-day lives, it is quite hard to think of anything that we don't use an online connection for in some way or another. From booking holidays, doing our grocery shopping, meeting the new Mr or Mrs Right in our lives, or finding a new job, the Internet connects it all. So, taking that thought a little further, can the Internet help us to earn a little extra cash when our flow isn't, well, flowing as fast as we would like?

Of course, it can!

The Internet is a fantastic place to start, and the beauty of all of it is that you can do it from the comfort of your armchair!

HOW
TO MAKE
MONEY
ONLINE

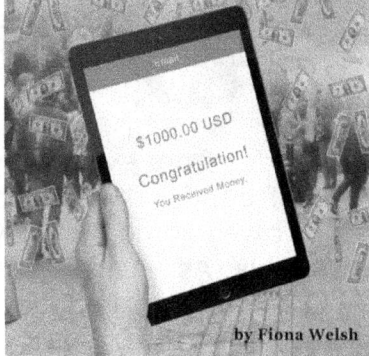

$1000.00 USD

Congratulation!

You Received Money.

by Fiona Welsh

<u>Keeping Your Children Safe</u> –
By Fiona Welsh (Self Help – Business)

Without a doubt, the most important and treasured things we have in our lives are our children. We give birth to them, we raise them, we worry about them, and we love them to the end of the world and back again. It is no surprise that when we see worrying events on the news, it first makes us think of our children.

We can't protect our kids from everything in life, and we can't shield them from the things that are going on around the globe, but we can do our very best to keep them as safe as possible. As a parent you will no doubt be very familiar with the thought that you want to wrap your children up in cotton wool and avert their eyes from anything that isn't Disney magical. Things can and do happen, but part of the solution is to know how to teach your children about safety in general, in the right way. Learning to show them that it is fine to explore, fine to live, but that being on the lookout for danger is vital.

So, how do you do that? How do you tread that fine line between living life and avoiding dangerous situations?

KEEPING YOUR
CHILDREN
SAFE

**INFORMATION AND ADVICE ON HOW TO PROTECT YOUR
CHILD AGAINST LIFE'S DARKER SIDE**

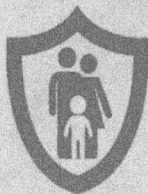

FIONA WELSH

We also have a selection of Adult Coloring Books to help relax pass the time and de-stress.
Beautiful Illustrations and puzzles in the back for your entertainment.

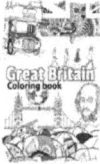

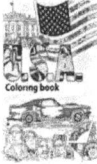

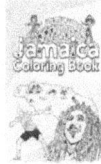

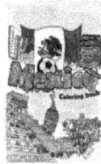

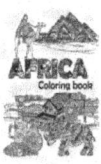

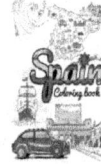

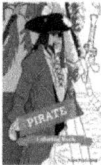

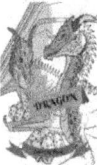

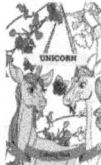

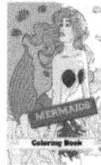

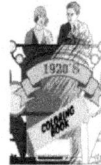

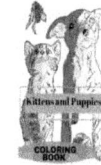

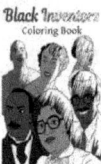

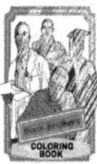

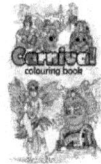

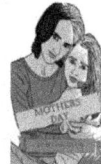

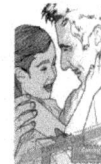

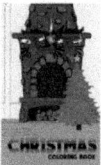

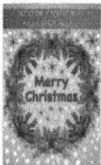

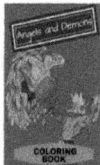

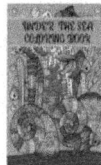

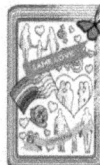

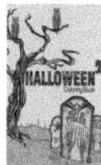

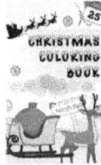

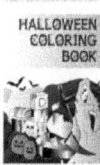

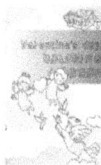

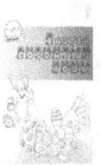

Visit **www.ArylaPublishing.com**
to find out about all new releases.

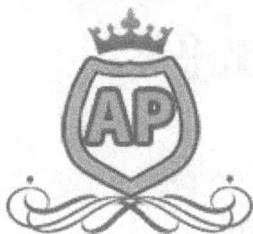

Follow us @arylapublishing on Twitter Instagram &
Facebook

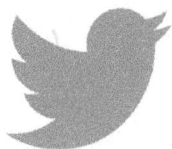

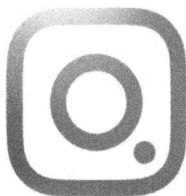

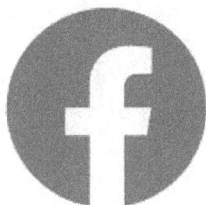

Search for Aryla Publishing on
▶ YouTube

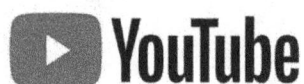

Check out our <u>Book Trailers</u>

<u>Subscribe</u> **to keep up to date with new releases!**

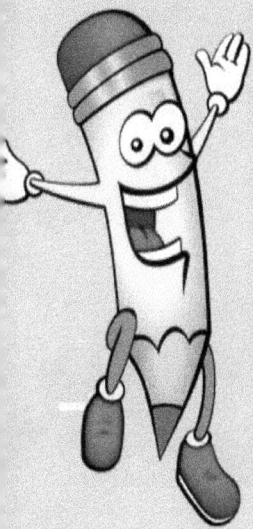

WE WOULD LOVE YOUR FEEDBACK

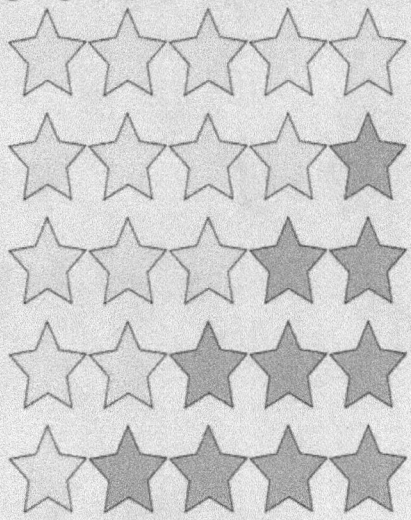

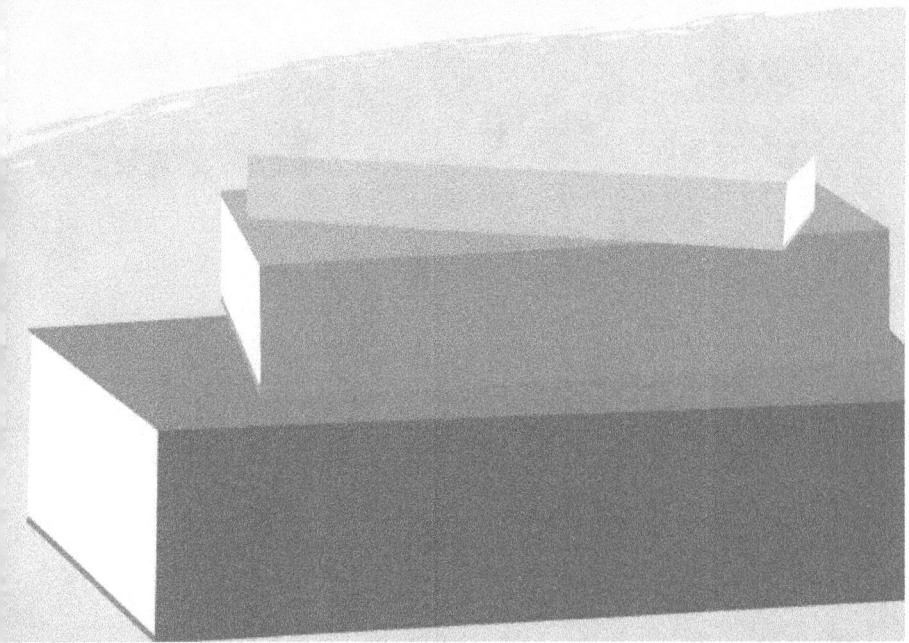

www.ingramcontent.com/pod-product-compliance
Lightning Source LLC
Chambersburg PA
CBHW060521280326
41933CB00014B/3059